Eye Anatomy
Handbook

H. A. Shah

Eye Anatomy Handbook

First Edition

Husnain A. Shah
MB BCh BAO
Honorary Medical Research Fellow
Department of Ophthalmology
Queen Elizabeth Hospital Birmingham

Table of Contents

Introduction

The purpose of this book is to provide a brief overview of the relevant anatomy for those interested in ophthalmology.

It is suitable for medical students and those starting ophthalmology training.

It can serve as an introduction to the Duke Elder examination and membership examination; however, it should not be your only resource for learning anatomy.

Chapter 1: Orbital Anatomy

Bones of the Calvarium

The bones of the calvarium are as follows:
- Frontal bone
- Temporal bone
- Parietal bone
- Occipital bone

Bones of the Cranial Base

The bones of the cranial base are as follows:
- Frontal bone
- Sphenoid bone
- Temporal bone
- Parietal bone
- Occipital bone
- Ethmoid bone

Bones of the Face

The bones of the face are as follows:
- Zygomatic bone
- Maxillary bone
- Nasal bone
- Lacrimal bone
- Mandibular bone

Pterion

The pterion is an H-shaped bony landmark where the frontal, parietal, temporal, and sphenoid bones join.

It is the weakest part of the skull.

The anterior division of the middle meningeal artery runs underneath the pterion.

As a consequence, trauma to the pterion can rupture the artery causing an epidural haematoma.

Sphenoid & Pterygoid

The sphenoid bone contains two pairs of 'wings': the greater wing and the lesser wing.

The greater wing contains the following foramina:
- Foramen rotundum
- Foramen ovale
- Foramen spinosum

The lesser wing contains the optic canal.

The optic canal contains the following structures:
- The optic nerve
- The ophthalmic artery
- Sympathetic fibres form the carotid plexus

Between the greater and lesser wings of the sphenoid is the superior orbital fissure.

Pterygopalatine Fossa

The contents of the pterygopalatine fossa are as follows:
- The pterygopalatine ganglion
- The maxillary artery
- The maxillary nerve (CN V$_2$)

Cranial Fossae

Anterior Cranial Fossa

The anterior cranial fossa contains the following:
- Foramen caecum
- Cribriform plate

Middle Cranial Fossa

The middle cranial fossa contains many important openings:
- Optic canal
- Superior orbital fissure
- Inferior orbital fissure
- Foramen rotundum
- Foramen ovale
- Foramen spinosum
- Foramen lacerum
- Carotid canal

Foramen Rotundum

The foramen rotundum transmits CN V$_2$.

Foramen Ovale

The foramen ovale transmits the following:
- **M**andibular nerve
- **M**otor root of the trigeminal nerve
- Accessory **m**eningeal nerve

Foramen Spinosum

The foramen spinosum transmits the following:
- Middle **meningeal** artery
- Middle **meningeal** vein
- **Meningeal** branch of the mandibular nerve

Posterior Cranial Fossa

The posterior cranial fossa contains the following openings:
- Foramen magnum
- Jugular foramen
- Hypoglossal canal
- Internal acoustic meatus
- Stylomastoid foramen

Paranasal Sinuses

The location of the sinuses relative to the orbit:

- The ethmoid and sphenoid sinuses is located medially

- The frontal sinus is located superiorly

- The maxillary sinus is located inferiorly

The four pairs of paranasal sinuses drain into the nasal cavity.

Openings of the Paranasal Sinuses

The posterior ethmoidal sinuses drain into the superior meatus.

The sphenoid sinus drains into the spheno-ethmoidal recess.

The frontal sinus, the maxillary sinus, and the anterior & middle ethmoidal sinuses drain into the middle meatus.

The nasolacrimal duct drains into the inferior meatus.

Head & Neck Blood Supply

Common Carotid Artery

The left common carotid artery arises from the aortic arch.

The right common carotid artery arises from the brachiocephalic artery.

The common carotid artery bifurcates at the level of the C4 vertebrae.

Carotid Sheath

The common carotid artery travels within the carotid sheath alongside the internal jugular vein and the vagus nerve.

External Carotid Artery

The external carotid artery has the following branches:
- Superior thyroid artery
- Lingual artery
- Facial artery
- Occipital artery
- Posterior auricular artery
- Ascending pharyngeal artery

The external carotid artery terminates as two branches:
- Superior temporal artery
- Maxillary artery

Internal Carotid Artery

The internal carotid artery has three branches:
- Ophthalmic artery
- Posterior communicating artery
- Anterior choroidal artery

Circle of Willis

The circle of Willis is composed of the following arteries:
- Anterior cerebral arteries
- Anterior communicating artery
- Internal carotid arteries
- Posterior cerebral arteries
- Posterior communicating artery

Ophthalmic Artery

The branches of the ophthalmic artery are as follows:
- Central retinal artery
- Long & short ciliary arteries
- Lacrimal artery
- Anterior ciliary arteries
- Supraorbital artery
- Ethmoid arteries
- Medial palpebral artery
- Dorsal nasal artery
- Supratrochlear artery

Venous Drainage: Head

The superior sagittal sinus drains posteriorly into the transverse sinus, which in turn joins the sigmoid sinus.

The great cerebral veins of Galen drain the deep cerebral veins into the straight sinus.

Venous Drainage: Orbit

The superior and inferior ophthalmic veins drain into the cavernous sinus.

The cavernous sinus drains into the superior and inferior petrosal sinuses.

The superior and inferior petrosal sinuses drain into the internal jugular veins via the sigmoid sinus.

Cavernous Sinus

The cavernous sinus contains the following structures:
- Lateral wall
  - oculomotor nerve
  - trochlear nerve
  - ophthalmic & maxillary branches of CN V
- Medial wall
  - abducens nerve
  - internal carotid artery
  - internal carotid plexus

Drainage of Cavernous Sinus

The cavernous sinus received blood from:
- Superior and inferior ophthalmic veins
- Spheno-parietal sinus
- Superficial middle cerebral veins
- Inferior cerebral veins

Pituitary Gland

The pituitary gland is located within the sella turcica within the sphenoid bone.

The pituitary gland is located below the optic chiasm.

The pituitary gland is drained by the cavernous sinus.

Bones of the Orbit

The orbit is composed of seven bones:

- Frontal
- Zygoma
- Maxillary
- Sphenoid
- Ethmoid
- Palatine
- Lacrimal

Orbital dimensions in the adult:

- The volume of the orbit is 30 millilitres.
- The orbit is shaped like a 'pear'.
- The orbital entrance is 35 mm in height; 45 mm in width.
- The orbital depth is 40-45 mm from entrance to apex.
- The orbit is widest 1 centimetre behind the anterior orbital margin.

The orbit contains no lymphatic vessels.

The orbit has four margins:

- The supraorbital margin is formed by the frontal bone.
- The medial margin is formed by frontal, lacrimal, and maxillary bones.
- The infraorbital margin is formed by the zygomatic and maxillary bones.
- The lateral margin is formed by the frontal and zygomatic bones.

The orbit has four walls:

- The roof is composed of the orbital plate of the frontal bone and lesser wing of sphenoid.
- The medial wall is composed of the frontal process of the maxilla, the lacrimal bone, the orbital plate of the ethmoid bone, and the body of the sphenoid bone.
- The floor is composed of the orbital plate of the zygomatic bone, the maxillary bone, and the palatine bone.
- The lateral wall is composed of the zygomatic bone, and the greater wing of sphenoid.

The ethmoid bone comprises the largest part of the medial orbital wall.

The lateral wall is the thickest wall of the orbit.

The lamina papyracea of the ethmoid bone is the weakest part of the orbit.

A blow-out fracture most commonly involves the orbital floor.

The lamina papyracea is the most common site of fracture following blunt trauma to the orbit.

The lateral orbital tubercle is located in the lateral orbital margin in the zygomatic bone.

The lateral orbital tubercle is the site of attachment for:
- Levator aponeurosis
- Lateral rectus check ligament
- Lockwood's ligament (suspensory ligament of the eyeball)
- Lateral canthal ligament
- Lacrimal gland fascia

Superior Orbital Fissure

The superior orbital fissure is located between the greater wing and the lesser wing of the sphenoid bone. It measures 22 millimetres in length.

Above the annulus of Zinn, the superior orbital fissure transmits the following structures:
- The lacrimal nerve of CN V_1
- The frontal nerve of CN V_1
- CN VI
- The superior ophthalmic vein

Within the annulus of Zinn, the superior orbital fissure transmits the following structures:
- Superior and inferior divisions of CN III
- The nasociliary branch of CN V_1
- The sympathetic roots of the ciliary ganglion
- CN VI

Inferior Orbital Fissure

The inferior orbital fissure transmits the following structures:
- The infraorbital and zygomatic branches of CN V_2
- The inferior ophthalmic vein

Chapter 2: Cranial Nerves

Olfactory Nerve

Cranial nerve I is also known as the olfactory nerve.

Fibres of CN I pass from the nasal cavity into the central nervous system through the cribriform plate of the ethmoid bone.

The olfactory tract runs beneath the frontal lobe of the brain.

The olfactory tract runs lateral to the gyrus rectus.

The Optic Nerve

Cranial nerve II is also known as the optic nerve.

There are four regions of the optic nerve
- The intraocular region, which measures 1 mm in length.
- The intra-orbital region, which measures 25 mm in length.
- The intra-canalicular region, which measures 4-10 mm in length.
- The intra-cranial region, which measures 10 mm in length.

The intra-cranial and intra-canalicular regions of the optic nerve have the widest diameter.

The intraorbital region of the optic nerve is the longest.

The blood supply to the optic nerve is as follows:
- The intraneural branches of the central retinal artery supply the intra-orbital region of the optic nerve.
- The pial branches of the ophthalmic artery supply the intra-canalicular region of the optic nerve.
- Branches of the internal carotid artery supply the intra-cranial region of the optic nerve.

Optic Disc

Optic disc measurements in adults:
1.76 mm horizontally; 1.92 mm vertically.

Lamina Cribrosa

The optic nerve head has four anatomical sub-divisions:
- The superficial nerve fibre layer
- The pre-laminar area
- The laminar area
- The retro-laminar area

The lamina cribrosa portion of the optic nerve head is composed of 10 connective tissue plates that are integrated with the sclera.

The lamina cribrosa is composed of type I and III collagen.

The optic nerve passes through the optic canal via the annulus of Zinn.

Optic nerve fibres are myelinated by oligodendrocytes.

Myelination of the optic nerve begins in the retro-laminar area.

Orbital Optic Nerve

Before entering the optic canal, the optic nerve is found supero-medial to the ophthalmic artery.

Within the orbit, the optic nerves are found infero-lateral to the ophthalmic artery.

The optic nerve passes superior to the cavernous sinus to join the optic chiasm.

Optic Chiasm

53% of optic nerve fibres cross at the optic chiasm.

Lateral Geniculate Nucleus

70% of the optic tract fibres go to the lateral geniculate nucleus.

Layers 1, 4, and 6 contain axons from the contralateral optic nerve.

Layers 2, 3, and 5 contain axons from the ipsilateral optic nerve.

Oculomotor Nerve

Cranial nerve III is also known as the oculomotor nerve.

Aneurysms that affect CN III commonly occur at the junction of the posterior communicating artery and the medial cerebral artery.

CN III runs along the lateral wall of the cavernous sinus.

CN III separates into the superior and inferior divisions after passing through the annulus of Zinn.

Parasympathetic fibres are found on the outside of CN III, and are typically the first to be affected by compressive aneurysms.

Oculomotor Nerve Nucleus

The nucleus of CN III is found in the rostral midbrain at the level of the superior colliculus.

Trochlear Nerve

Cranial nerve IV is also known as the trochlear nerve.

CN IV has the longest intracranial course of the cranial nerves.

The nucleus of CN IV is found in the caudal midbrain at the level of the inferior colliculus.

CN IV is found on the lateral wall of the cavernous sinus. CN IV is located outside the intermuscular cone; therefore it is typically not affected by retro-bulbar anaesthetics.

Trigeminal Nerve

CN V is also known as the trigeminal nerve.

Trigeminal Nerve Nuclei

CN V has four nuclei:
- Mesencephalic nucleus
- Main sensory nucleus
- Spinal nucleus
- Motor nucleus

The mesencephalic nucleus mediates proprioception to the facial and extraocular muscles. It is found at the level of the midbrain.

The main sensory nucleus provides light touch from the skin and mucous membranes. It is found at the level of the pons.

The spinal nucleus provides pain and temperature sensation to the face. It is found at the level of the medulla.

The motor nucleus innervates the following muscle groups:
- Muscles of mastication (pterygoids, and masseters temporalis)
- Tensor tympani
- Tensor veli palatine
- Mylohyoid
- Anterior belly of digastric

CN V is divided into three branches:

- V_1 also known as the ophthalmic nerve
- V_2 also known as the maxillary nerve
- V_3 also known as the mandibular nerve

Ophthalmic Nerve Divisions

CN V_1 is divided into three (further) branches:

- Lacrimal nerve
- Frontal nerve
- Nasociliary nerve

CN V_1 & V_2 are found on the lateral wall of the cavernous sinus.

Frontal Nerve Divisions

The frontal nerve divides into the supra-orbital and supra-trochlear nerves.

The supra-trochlear nerve exits the orbit 17 mm from the midline; the supra-orbital nerve exits 27 mm from the midline.

These nerves innervate the mediate portion of the upper eyelid and the conjunctiva.

The lacrimal nerve innervates the lacrimal gland and the nearby conjunctiva and skin.

CN V_2 divides into three main branches:

- Infra-orbital nerve

- Zygomatic nerve
- Superior alveolar nerve

The infra-orbital nerve divides (further) into three main branches:
- Inferior palpebral branch of the lower eyelid
- Nasal branch
- Superior labial branch

Long & Short Ciliary Nerves

Long ciliary nerves carry:
- Sensory fibres from the ciliary body, iris, and cornea
- Sympathetic innervation to the dilator muscle of the iris

Short ciliary nerves carry:
- Sensation to the globe
- Parasympathetics to the sphincter and ciliary muscles

Abducens Nerve

Cranial nerve VI is also known as the abducens nerve.

The nucleus of CN VI is found anterior to the fourth ventricle in the caudal pons.

CN VI is most susceptible to stretch injury from raised intracranial pressure due to its tortuous course.

CN VI is located adjacent to the medial wall of the cavernous sinus, below the carotid artery.

Facial Nerve

Cranial nerve VII is also known as the facial nerve.

The nucleus of CN VII is in the caudal pons, adjacent to the nucleus of CN VI.

CN VII emerges from the cerebello-pontine angle.

CN VII supplies the muscles of facial expression.

Chapter 3: Extra-Ocular Muscles

The Extra-Ocular Muscles

The extraocular muscles are responsible for the movements of the eyeball.

They consist of two types of muscle fibres: fast-twitch fibres, and slow-twitch fibres.

Compared to skeletal muscle they contain more connective tissue; they contain more nerve fibres; and they are better vascularised.

Rectus Muscle Origin

The rectus muscles originate from the common tendinous ring, which is also known as the annulus of Zinn.

It is located in the posterior orbit.

Rectus Muscle Tendon Length

The medial rectus has the shortest tendon: 3.7 mm.

The lateral rectus has the longest tendon: 8.8 mm.

Rectus Muscle Insertions

The tendons of the rectus muscles insert into the sclera behind the limbus at varying distances.

The medial rectus inserts 5.5 mm from the limbus.

The inferior rectus inserts 6.5 mm from the limbus.

The lateral rectus inserts 6.9 mm from the limbus.

The superior rectus inserts 7.7 mm from the limbus.

Muscle Actions

The actions of the extraocular muscles can be categorised as primary, secondary, and tertiary.

Primary Actions

The primary action of the medial rectus is adduction.

The primary action of the lateral rectus is abduction.

The primary action of the inferior rectus is depression.

The primary action of the superior rectus is elevation.

The primary action of the inferior oblique is extorsion.

The primary action of the superior oblique is intorsion.

Secondary Actions

The secondary action of the inferior rectus is extorsion.

The secondary action of the superior rectus is intorsion.

The secondary action of the inferior oblique is elevation.

The secondary action of the superior oblique is depression.

Tertiary Actions

The tertiary action of the inferior rectus is adduction.

The tertiary action of the superior rectus is adduction.

The tertiary action of the inferior oblique is abduction.

The tertiary action of the superior oblique is abduction.

Chapter 4: Eyelids

The palpebral fissure is the space between the upper and lower eyelids.

Dimensions of the adult palpebral fissure:
- 8-11 mm in height; 27-30 mm in width.

Eyelid Structures

Eyelid structures from superficial to deep:
- Thin skin
- Subcutaneous tissue
- Orbicularis oculi fibres
- Orbital septum / tarsal plates
- Levator (in upper lid)
- Conjunctiva

Eyelid Muscles

The levator palpebrae superioris is capable of 15 mm of upper eyelid elevation.

The palpebral fissure can be widened an additional 2 mm by the action of the frontalis muscle.

Muscles of retraction of the lower eyelid:
- Capsulopalpebral fascia
- Inferior tarsal muscle

Glands

- Meibomian glands are holocrine glands which sit within the tarsal plate and secrete the lipid component of the tear film.
- Sebaceous glands of Zeis open into the ciliary follicles.
- Glands of Moll are modified apocrine sweat glands.

Grey Line

- The grey line of the eyelid corresponds to the muscle of Riolan.
- Anterior to the grey line are the eyelashes.
- Posterior to the grey line are the Meibomian glands.

Conjunctiva

Conjunctiva can be divided into three divisions:
- Palpebral conjunctiva
- Bulbar conjunctiva
- Forniceal conjunctiva

Parts of the orbicularis oculi muscle
- Orbital portion
- Pre-septal portion
- Pre-tarsal portion

The pre-septal and pre-tarsal portions of the orbicularis oculi are responsible for spontaneous and reflex blinking.

The pre-tarsal portion of the orbicularis oculi is uniquely responsible for tear drainage.

Orbital Fascia

The tarsal plates are attached to the orbital margin by the medial and lateral palpebral ligaments.

The upper and lower tarsi are 29 mm wide and 1 mm thick.

The upper tarsus is 11 mm in height.

The lower tarsus is 4 mm in height.

Eyelid Vessels

The facial artery becomes the angular artery as it passes upward and lateral to the nose.

The marginal arterial arcade is the arterial supply near the eyelid margin.

The superior peripheral arcade is the arterial supply found near the upper eyelid crease.

The superficial venous drainage system of the eyelid is to the internal and external jugular veins.

The deep venous drainage system of the eyelid is to the cavernous sinus.

Eyelid Lymphatics

The lymphatics to the eyelids:
- The medial group that drains into the submandibular lymph nodes.
- The lateral group that drains into the superficial pre-auricular lymph nodes.

Chapter 5: Lacrimal Anatomy

The lacrimal glands perform exocrine secretion of aqueous content.

The Krause and Wolfring glands perform exocrine secretion of aqueous content.

The Meibomian glands perform holocrine secretion of lipid content.

The Zeis glands perform holocrine secretion of lipid content.

The Moll glands perform apocrine secretion of sweat content.

The goblet cells perform holocrine secretion of mucous content.

The lacrimal gland is divided in two by the levator aponeurosis.

The lacrimal gland ducts empty into the conjunctival fonix.

The lacrimal puncta measure 0.3 mm in diameter.

The superior lacrimal puncta are located more medially than the inferior lacrimal puncta.

The inferior punctum is 6.5 mm from the medial canthus.

The superior punctum is 6 mm from the medial canthus.

The nasolacrimal duct drains into the inferior meatus of the nose.

Chapter 6: Conjunctiva

The Conjunctiva

Function
The conjunctiva serves a number of functions:

- It provides lubrication via mucous and tears
- It presents a mechanical barrier to micro-organisms
- It aids immune surveillance

Anatomy
The conjunctiva is a thin, transparent mucus membrane.

It covers the sclera and lines the inside of the eyelids.

It is nourished by tiny blood vessels.

Caruncle
The lacrimal caruncle is a highly vascular nodule of modified skin.

It contains large nests of accessory lacrimal and sebaceous glandular tissue.

It is debatably a vestigial organ.

Plica Semilunaris
The plica semilunaris is located lateral and slightly inferior to the caruncle.

It is a small fold of bulbar conjunctiva.

It is highly vascular, and rich in goblet cells and immunocompetent cells.

It may facilitate lateral eye movement.

Structure

The conjunctiva is typically divided in three parts:

- The palpebral conjunctiva
- The bulbar conjunctiva
- The forniceal conjunctiva

Palpebral Conjunctiva

The palpebral or tarsal conjunctiva lines the under-surface of eyelids.

Bulbar Conjunctiva

The bulbar conjunctiva covers the sclera.

It contains goblet cells.

It is tightly bound to sclera by Tenon's capsule.

It moves with eye-ball movement.

Forniceal Conjunctiva

The forniceal conjunctiva is located at the junction between the eyelid and eyeball.

It permits free rotation of the eyeball.

It is loosely attached to the fascial sheaths of the levator palpabrae superioris and the rectus muscles.

Protective Cells

The conjunctival epithelium contains a number of protective cells:

- Goblet cells, which secrete mucous
- Melanocytes, which release melanosomes
- Langerhan's cells, which are antigen-presenting cells
- Intraepithelial lymphocytes, which increase during inflammation

Nerve Supply

The bulbar conjunctiva is supplied by ciliary nerves.

The superior palpebral conjunctiva and superior fornix are supplied by branches of ophthalmic nerve.

The inferior palpebral conjunctiva and inferior fornix are supplied by branches of the ophthalmic nerve, and by the infraorbital nerve.

Tear Film

The Tear Film
The tear film is composed of three layers:

- The outer lipid layer
- The middle aqueous layer
- The inner mucin layer

Lipid Layer
The lipid layer contains oils.

It is secreted by Meibomian glands.

It coats the aqueous layer.

It serves as a hydrophobic barrier.

It prevents tears spilling.

Aqueous Layer
The aqueous layer contains water, proteins and lysozyme.

It is secreted by the lacrimal gland.

It promotes the spreading of the tear film.

It protects against infection

It promotes osmotic regulation.

Mucin Layer

The mucin layer coats the cornea.

It is produced by goblet cells.

It forms a hydrophilic layer.

It allows for the even distribution of tears.

Chapter 7: Cornea

The Cornea

The cornea is the outermost layer of the eye.

It performs the majority of the refraction of light.

It has a fixed curvature.

It represents a barrier to infection.

It functions as a filter to UV light, which serves to protect the lens and the retina.

Anatomy

The cornea is composed of five microscopic layers:

- Epithelium
- Bowman's layer
- Stroma
- Descemet's membrane
- Endothelium

Corneal Epithelium

The corneal epithelium is a stratified, squamous, non-keratinised epithelium.

It is composed of 5-6 cell layers.

It contains three cells types:

- Superficial cells
- Wing cells
- Basal cells

Epithelial Layers

Superficial Cells

The superficial cell layer measures 2-3 cells in thickness.

Superficial cells are flat cells with horizontal nuclei.

They are attached to each other via desmosomes.

They contain microvilli and microplicae on their surface, which help to stabilise the pre-corneal tear film.

They are lost with age.

Wing Cells

The middle zone of the corneal epithelium consists of wing cells.

These are polyhedral in shape.

They attach to each other via desmosomes.

Basal Cells

Basal cells represent the deepest cells.

These are tall and columnar.

They consist of a single layer resting on a basal lamina.

They attach to the basement membrane via hemidesmosomes.

Corneal Limbus

The corneal limbus represents the border between the cornea and the sclera.

It is composed of radial epithelial folds, known collectively as the palisades of Vogt.

These palisades are the site of the limbal stem cells.

Limbal Stem Cells

Limbal stem cells are responsible for the regeneration of corneal epithelium.

They are poorly-differentiated, and have a high capacity for self-renewal.

Injury may result in stem cell failure. As a consequence, there can be opacification of the cornea.

Bowman's Layer

Bowman's layer is located immediately beneath the basement membrane of corneal epithelium.

It consists of modified acellular stroma.

It measures 8-12 μm in thickness.

It is composed of types I, III, V & VI collagen.

It does not regenerate after injury.

Stroma

The corneal stroma is composed of dense, regular connective tissue.

It constitutes 90% of the cornea.

It measures approx. 500 μm in thickness.

It contains predominantly type I collagen.

It is transparent due to regular collagen fibril spacing.

It contains no blood vessels or lymphatic vessels.

Descemet's Membrane

Descemet's membrane is a thin layer between the posterior stroma and the endothelium.

It measures 8-12 μm in thickness.

It is a modified basement membrane.

It is rich in type IV collagen.

Endothelium

The corneal endothelium is a monolayer of mitochondria-rich cells.

It regulates fluid and solute transport between aqueous humour and corneal stroma.

It maintains hydration and thus transparency.

Endothelial cells of the cornea have a low regenerative capacity.

Endothelial cell density diminishes with age.

Nerve Supply

The cornea is supplied by the long ciliary nerves.

Damage to the corneal epithelium and terminal nerve ending causes severe pain.

Chapter 8: Sclera

The Sclera

The sclera is a fibrous connective tissue, which forms the outer part of the eye.

It protects the eye from light and gives the eye its shape.

It attaches to the optic nerve posteriorly.

It is thin in children and patients with glaucoma, and becomes thicker with age.

It has significant sensory innervation.

It is the sight of insertion of the extraocular muscles. Consequently, pain caused by inflammation is made worse with eye movement.

Scleral Apertures

The sclera is pierced by **three groups** of small apertures:

- **Anterior apertures** are located at the insertion of the recti muscles and are for branches of the anterior ciliary arteries.
- **Middle apertures** are located approx. 4 mm posterior to the equator of the eye and are for the exit of the vortex veins.
- **Posterior apertures** are small and numerous and are located around the optic nerve. They transmit the long and the short posterior ciliary nerves and vessels.

Sclera Thickness

The sclera is **thickest** posteriorly, measuring 1mm

At the equator it measures 0.6 mm

The sclera is **thinnest** at the insertion of the rectus muscles, measuring 0.3 mm.

Scleral Blood Supply

The scleral blood supply is derived from the anterior and posterior ciliary arteries, which branch from the ophthalmic artery.

Structure of the Sclera

The sclera consists of three layers:

- The episclera
- The scleral stroma
- The lamina fusca

Layers of the Sclera

Episclera

The episclera is the outermost layer consisting of loose connective tissue anteriorly connecting sclera and conjunctiva.

It is connected to the fascial sheath of the eye ball (Tenon's capsule) by fine strands of tissue.

Anteriorly, it has a rich blood supply (anterior ciliary arteries) forming a plexus between the extrinsic muscle insertions and the corneo-scleral junction.

Episcleral thickness decreases towards the back of the eye

Scleral Stroma

Dense fibrous tissue intermingled with fine elastic fibres.

Consists of collagen fibres (type I and III), which range in diameter from 28 to 280 µm.

Bundles of fibres are arranged irregularly.

A few elongated fibroblasts are found between the collagen bundles. Occasional melanocytes can also be seen.

Lamina Fusca

The lamina fusca is the innermost layer of the sclera,

It is faintly brown (melanocytes), thin, and irregular.

It is separated from the external surface of the choroid by the perichoroidal (suprachoridal) space.

Fine collagen fibres connect the lamina fusca with the choroid, forming a weak attachment between the sclera and the choroid.

Nerve Supply

The nerve supply to the anterior sclera are two long ciliary nerves.

The nerve supply to the posterior sclera are the short ciliary nerves.

Blood Supply

The blood supply to the anterior sclera is the anterior ciliary artery.

The blood supply to the posterior sclera are the long and short posterior ciliary arteries.

Lamina Cribrosa

The lamina cribrosa is a mesh-like structure that permits the passage of the optic nerve through the sclera.

Matrix Proteins

The sclera consists of the following matrix proteins:

- Collagens I and III
- Proteoglycans combined with hyaluronic acid

Chapter 9: Uvea

The Uvea

The uvea consists of the choroid, ciliary body, and iris.

Chapter 10: Iris

The Iris

The iris is a thin, pigmented diaphragm.

Located in the middle of the iris is the pupil.

It measures 12 mm in diameter and 37 mm in circumference.

It separates the anterior chamber from the posterior chamber.

The size of the pupil in controlled by two muscles: the sphincter pupillae and the dilator pupillae.

Histology

The iris consists of four layers

- Anterior border
- Stroma
- Dilator pupillae
- Posterior pigment epithelium

Anterior border

The anterior border is composed of a modified stroma with areas of deficiency (known as crypts).

Stroma

The iris stroma is composed of loosely-arranged connective tissue: collagen types I and III.

The sphincter pupillae is innervated by the postganglionic parasympathetic fibres of the short ciliary nerves.

Dilator pupillae

The dilator pupillae extends only to the outer margin of the sphincter pupillae centrally.

It is innervated by non-myelinated sympathetic fibres (nasociliary and long ciliary nerves).

Posterior pigment epithelium

The posterior pigment epithelium is a highly-pigmented cuboidal epithelium. The posterior epithelial layer forms a series of radially arranged furrows.

Blood Supply

The iris is supplied by the major & minor arterial circles.

Pupil function

The pupil can dilate (mydriasis) and constrict (miosis).

This can change the magnitude off light entering the eye.

During accommodation the pupil constricts and reduces spherical aberration.

Chapter 11: Ciliary Body

The Ciliary Body

The ciliary body consists of a 5-6mm ring of tissue, which extends from the scleral spur anteriorly to the ora serrata posteriorly.

The ciliary body is wider temporally than nasally.

It forms a triangle on cross section with the base towards the anterior chamber and the apex blending with the choroid posteriorly.

Anatomically it is divided into two parts:

Anterior functional part: pars plicata.

Posterior non-functional part: pars plana.

The ciliary body projects 70 ciliary processes.

Histology

The ciliary body consists of three layers: the epithelium, stroma, and muscle.

Ciliary Epithelium

The ciliary epithelium is composed of two layers of cubical cells: one pigmented; one non-pigmented.

Theses layers are arranged with their apices facing one another.

The non-pigmented inner layer lines the posterior chamber and the pigmented outer layer faces the stroma of the ciliary body.

The non-pigmented layer is the anterior continuation of the neural retina.

The pigmented layer is the anterior continuation of the RPE.

Stroma

The stroma is a loose connective tissue, rich in blood vessels and melanocytes.

Muscle

Muscle composes the bulk of the ciliary body substance.

It consists of three layers:

- Longitudinal (outermost)
- Oblique
- Circular (innermost)

Blood Supply

The arterial blood supply to the choroid is as follows:

- The long posterior ciliary and anterior ciliary arteries.
- Muscular and recurrent choroidal branches form the vascular plexus of the ciliary processes.

The venous drainage of the choroid is as follows:

- Vortex veins (majority)
- Anterior ciliary veins (minority)

Nerve Supply

The ciliary body is primarily innervated by preganglionic parasympathetic fibres from the Edinger-Westphal nucleus in the midbrain.

Function

The ciliary body serves numerous functions.

Accommodation

Cciliary muscle contraction leads to laxity in the zonular fibres which allows the lens to obtain a more spherical shape and increases its refractive power.

Aqueous Production

70 ciliary processes which are delicate protrusions of vascular connective tissue lined by bilaminar cuboidal neuroectoderm. Aqueous secretion is via the inner non-pigmented layer of the ciliary body. This layer has tight junctions at its apical surface.

Zonular Production

Occurs via the non-pigmented cuboidal epithelial cells of the pars plana.

Glycosaminoglycan Production

The posterior ciliary body secretes GAG's like extracellular components such as hyalouronic acid into the vitreous body.

Chapter 12: Choroid

The choroid is the vascular layer of the eye lying between the retina and the sclera.

It provides oxygen and nourishment to the outer layers of the retina.

It is firmly attached to the sclera at the edges of the optic nerve.

Structure

The choroid consists of four layers

- Haller's layer: outermost layer of the choroid consisting of larger diameter blood vessels.
- Sattler's layer: layer of medium diameter blood vessels.
- Choriocapillaris: layer of capillaries, high density at macula with wider bore.
- Bruch's membrane: innermost layer of the choroid.

The choroid receives its blood supply from the short posterior ciliary artery and anterior ciliary vessels.

The choroid contains melanocytes, which absorb excess light that penetrates the retina, thus preventing reflection.

It is supplied by long and short ciliary nerves

The long ciliary nerve is a branch of the nasociliary nerve, which is a branch of ophthalmic division of the trigeminal nerve.

The short ciliary nerves branch off the ciliary ganglion.

Bruch's Membrane

Bruch's membrane consists of five layers:

- The basement membrane of RPE
  The inner collagenous zone
- The middle elastic layer
- The outer collagenous zone
- The basement membrane of the choriocapillaris

The retinal pigment epithelium transports metabolic waste from the across Bruch's membrane to the choroid.

Chapter 13: Lens

The Lens

The lens is a transparent, biconvex structure located behind the iris.

In the adult, it measures 10x4 mm.

It helps to refract light to focus on the retina.

Its curvature is controlled by the ciliary muscles.

Structure

The crystalline lens is composed of 4 layers:

- Capsule
- Subcapsular epithelium
- Cortex
- Nucleus

Capsule

The capsule is generated by the cells of the subcapsular epithelium.

It is a clear and elastic basal membrane-like structure that keeps it under constant tension (3-20 μm).

It consists of 40 lamellae (40 nm each in thickness).

It consists of type IV collagen.

Nucleus

The nucleus is the innermost part of the lens and is surrounded by the cortex.

It originates from cells that have lost their nuclei and become packed by crystallins to form lens fibers.

Crystallins account for 60% of the mass of lens fibres.

Mature lens fibres are hexagonal in shape and can measure up to 12 mm in length.

Lens fibres are nucleated in the soft, outer cortex of the lens.

As new lens fibres are added to the periphery of the cortex, lens fibres located deeper in the cortex lose their nuclei and become part of the harder nucleus of the lens.

The lens functions as one cell due to numerous gap junctions, and inter-digitation of plasma membrane.

Zonular Fibres

The lens is suspended within the eye by suspensory fibrous strands called zonules of Zinn, which attach at one end to the lens capsule and at the other end to the epithelial layer of the ciliary body around the inside of the eye.

These fibres hold the lens in place.

Characteristics

The average adult human lens is about 4-5 mm thick and has a diameter of about 9-10 mm. Its thickness can be adjusted by surrounding muscles, and crystallins are its main protein building blocks.

Composition

Crystallins are arranged in approximately 20,000 thin concentric layers.

The refractive index of the lens ranges from approx. 1.406 (central layers) to 1.36 in less dense cortex of the lens.

This index gradient enhances the optical power of the lens.

Function

The function of the lens is to change the focal distance of the eye to allow focusing on objects at various distances. This process is called accommodation.

With age, the lens gradually hardens, which reduces the ability to accommodate (8 diopters at age 40, 1-2 diopters at age 60).

The refractive power of the lens in situ is approx. 15 dioptres.

Chapter 14: Retina

The Retina

The retina represents the innermost layer of the eye.

It is where optical images are transformed into neural impulses.

The retina can be divided into two parts:

- The inner neurosensory retina
- The outer retinal pigment epithelium (RPE)

These two layers are adherent due to negative pressure, viscous proteoglycans and electrostatic forces.

The retina is continuous anteriorly with the ciliary processes and posterior iris surface, and posteriorly continuous with the optic nerve.

The retina is bound externally by Bruch's membrane and internally by the vitreous.

It has a surface area measuring 1250 mm^2.

Regions

The retina can be divided into 7 areas:

- The posterior pole
- Macula lutea
- Fovea centralis
- Optic disc
- Peripheral retina
- Ora serra
- Foveal avascular zone

Posterior Pole

The posterior pole (area centralis) is located between the superior and inferior retinal arcades. It represents a cone-rich region with more than one layer of ganglion cells.

Macula Lutea

The macula lutea /fovea measures 1.5 mm in diameter and is located 3mm lateral to optic disc.

The macula is rich in the yellow xanthophyll carotenoid pigment, which helps to block UV light.

Fovea Centralis

The fovea centralis/foveola measures 0.35 mm in diameter. Here no rods are found but is marked by maximal cone density. This area is avascular and relies on the choriocapillaris for nutrition.

Optic Disc

The optic disc is located 3 mm medial to macula, and corresponds to physiological blind spot.

Peripheral Retina

The peripheral retina is the remainder of retina outside the posterior pole and is rich in rod photoreceptors.

Ora Serrata

The ora serrata is the anterior scalloped region of retina.

Foveal Avascular Zone

The foveal avascular zone (FAZ) is 0.5mm in diameter.

Layers of the Retina

Internal limiting membrane

Nerve fibre layer

Ganglion cell layer

Inner plexiform layer

Inner nuclear layer

Outer plexiform layer

Outer nuclear layer

External limiting membrane

Photoreceptors

RPE

Chapter 15: RPE

Retinal Pigment Epithelium

The retinal pigment epithelium is a continuous monolayer of hexagonal cuboidal cells.

It measures 4.2-6.1 million cells.

It is more columnar in shape in the central retina and more flattened in the peripheral retina.

The cells of the RPE are joined near their apical margins by tight junctions, which help to form the outer blood-retinal barrier.

RPE Function

The RPE serves many functions:

- Essential for photoreceptor health
- Vitamin A metabolism
- Phagocytosis of photoreceptor outer segments
- Light absorption
- Secretion of the photoreceptor extracellular matrix
- Active transport of materials between the choriocapillaris and the sub-retinal space
- Decreasing light scatter within the eye

Photoreceptors

The human retina contains two types of photoreceptor: rods and cones.

Rods number 120 million and are most abundant in the periphery. Cones number 6 million and are most abundant in the macula.

Rods are important for contrast, brightness, and motion.

Cones are important for fine resolution, spatial resolution and colour vision.

Blood Supply

The retina is supplied by the retinal blood vessels and the choroid.

Chapter 16: Vitreous

The Vitreous

The vitreous cavity contains 80% of the volume of the eye.

It weights approx 3.9 g

It is composed 98% of water.

It has a refractive index of 1.33

The viscous properties of the vitreous allow the eye to return to its normal shape if compressed.

The viscosity of the vitreous is 2-4 times that of water.

It is surrounded by a thin membrane known as the hyaloid membrane.

No blood vessels penetrate the vitreous body; therefore its nutrition must be carried on by vessels of the retina and ciliary processes.

Composition of the Vitreous

The vitreous is composed of the following:

- Water (98%)
- Collagen II fibrils
- Hyaluronic acid
- Hyalocytes
- Inorganic salts
- Glucose
- Ascorbic acid

Chapter 17: Embryology

Neuroectoderm

The neuroectoderm is the origin of the following tissues:

- Retina: neurosensory and RPE
- Epithelial lining of the iris and ciliary body
- Optic nerves

Surface Ectoderm

The surface ectoderm is the origin of the following tissues:

- Lens
- Corneal epithelium
- Conjunctival epithelium
- Lacrimal gland
- Nasolacrimal system
- Meibomian glands

Neural Crest

The neural crest is the origin of the following tissues:

- Sclera
- Iris stroma
- Corneal stroma and endothelium
- Trabecular meshwork and Schlemm's canal
- Extraocular muscles
- Ciliary muscle
- Connective tissue and bony structure of the orbit

Mesoderm

The mesoderm is the origin of the following tissues:

- Extraocular muscles
- Endothelial lining of blood vessels of the eye
- Blood vessels in the sclera and choroid
- Sclera
- Vitreous
- Suspensory fibres
- Angle outflow apparatus

Suggested Resources

Anatomy

Clinical Anatomy of the Eye, 2nd Edition
The Eye: Basic Sciences in Practice, 4th Edition

Duke Elder

The Duke Elder Exam of Ophthalmology: A Comprehensive Guide for Success

FRCOphth Online Question Banks

eFRCOphth
eyeQ

Printed in Great Britain
by Amazon

45239909R00046